Organic Body Sprays:
Top 35 Homemade Spray Recipes For Body

The information herein is offered for informational purposes solely, and is universal as so. The presentation of the information is without contract or any type of guarantee assurance.

The trademarks that are used are without any consent, and the publication of the trademark is without permission or backing by the trademark owner. All trademarks and brands within this book are for clarifying purposes only and are the owned by the owners themselves, not affiliated with this document.

Table of content

Introduction

Keeping cool in the summer can seem almost impossible, especially if you are spending a lot of time outside. Summer can also be a bit difficult if you live in an area where you have to deal with severe weather which often leads to power outages and very hot people.

Many people find relief by swimming or hang out under the sprinkler, but what if you don't want to get wet or if you work at a job where you have to be outside all day long?

Working outside can be almost unbearable as can working in a factory that is not air conditioned, however, there are things that you can do to relieve some of the heat. In this book, we are going to go over 35 cooling sprays that you can make right at home and take with you all of the time so that you are able to stay cool.

On top of this, you are going to find that many of these cooling sprays have other benefits besides helping keep you cool. Many of the cooling sprays are going to help you reduce wrinkles, fine lines, age spots, red spots, reduce acne, or simply help you reduce your stress levels.

All of the cooling sprays that you will find in this book are made out of all-natural, healthy ingredients that are going to provide many benefits to your skin. As we work through each of the cooling sprays, you will learn all of their benefits, as well as any warnings that come along with them.

It is important to know that as you work through this book and create these cooling sprays that you should only be using the finest of ingredients. You should always make sure that you are using food grade essential oils as well as other quality ingredients because you are going to be using these sprays on your face and body. If you use low-quality essential oils or other ingredients, you will risk rashes, burning, irritation, as well as other skin issues.

You should also test out all of the ingredients on a small patch of skin before mixing them and creating the sprays, especially if you do not know how you are going to react to them or if you have sensitive skin.

Chapter 1 – Natural Cooling Sprays

1. Aloe Vera Gel Cooling Spray

You will need:

3 tablespoons of high-quality Aloe Vera gel

3 tablespoons of witch hazel

5 drops of Peppermint Essential Oil

Directions:

Mix the Aloe Vera gel and the witch hazel in a small mist bottle and shake well. Add one drop of Peppermint Essential Oil at a time, shake well and spritz on the face to test the potency. Do not add more than 5 drops of Peppermint Essential Oil. This is important because, the Essential Oil is very potent and if you add too much, it will cause a cold burning sensation where you use it.

It is also very important to know that this cooling spray is best used on oily skin because witch hazel and Aloe Vera gel can cause your skin to dry out. This can cause problems if you already have dry skin. This is also a great cooling spray if you have been sweating because it will dry up all of the oils, however, even if you do have oily skin, this mist should not be used more than three times per day.

2. Simple Cooling Spray

You will need:

5 drops of Lavender Essential oil

1 drop of Peppermint Essential Oil

1 cup of distilled water.

Directions:

Mix all of the ingredients in a spray bottle and shake well. This is a great spray to use on your arms, legs, and back. When you use this spray on your face, make sure that you do not get it in your eyes.

3. Cooling spray to soothe a sunburn

You will need:

20 drops of Lavender Essential oil

1 ounce of distilled water

Directions:

Mix the two ingredients in a spray bottle and shake well before spraying on the sunburn. You can use as often as is needed to soothe the sunburn.

4. Hot Flash Cooling Spray

You will need:

1 drop of Rose Essential Oil

3 drops of Roman Chamomile Essential Oil

5 drops of Lavender Essential oil

2 ounces of distilled water

Directions:

Place all of the ingredients in a spray bottle and shake well before each use. Use as needed to help you cool down when you are having a hot flash.

Many people search for relief when they are having a hot flash, going as far as sticking their head in the freezer, however, when you use this cooling spray, you will no longer have to suffer when those hot flashes show up

5. Super Cooling Spray

You will need:

4 drops of Clary Sage Essential Oil

3 drops of Roman Chamomile Essential Oil

3 drops of Geranium Essential Oil

2 drops of Cypress Essential oil

1 drop of Peppermint Essential Oil

1 cup of distilled water

Directions:

Begin by mixing all of the essential oils in your spray bottle and then add in the cup of distilled water. Shake well before each use. Use this cooling spray whenever you need to cool down.

6. Green Tea Cooling Spray

You will need:

2 ounces of strongly brewed Green tea

2 tablespoons of Aloe Vera gel

5 drops of Peppermint Essential Oil

Directions:

Begin by placing 2 ounces of water in a ceramic cup along with 1 Green tea bag. Place in the microwave for one minute and then allow the tea to steep for 20 minutes.

Place the 2 tablespoons of Aloe Vera gel in your spray bottle (should be a spray bottle that is about 2 ounces). Pour the tea into the spray bottle until the bottle is about ¾ of the way filled. Next, add in your 5 drops of Peppermint Essential Oil.

As with the first cooling spray in this book, you may want to add one drop at a time and test it on your face as adding too much Peppermint Essential oil can cause a cold burning sensation.

Shake well before each use and use as needed. This is a great cooling spray that can be used on all types of skin because the Peppermint Essential oil does not dry out the skin and the Green tea actually helps to keep the skin smooth and soft.

It is important to know that if this cooling spray is left to sit for too long, the tea will go bad, however, most people find that they are using the bottle long before they have to worry about the tea going bad.

7. Hydrating Cooling Body Spray

You will need:

.25 ounces of grapeseed oil

3 drops of Litsea Cubeba Essential Oil

2 drops of rose absolute

.25 ounces of solubilizer (carrier oil such as coconut oil)

1 teaspoon of silk peptides

.07 ounces of vegetable glycerin

100 ml of Aloe Vera juice this is not Aloe Vera gel

Any broad-spectrum preservative

Directions:

Begin by measuring out the grapeseed oil as well as the essential oils and placing them in a 3.3-ounce spray bottle. Add the solubilizer next, followed by 1/3 of the Aloe Vera juice. Place the lid on top and swirl the bottle to combine the ingredients.

Take the lid off and add in the rest of the ingredients including the rest of the Aloe Vera juice. Place the lid on and shake well. Spritz this on your skin to not only cool, but to hydrate as well.

8. Repairing Cooling Spray

You will need:

1 bag of Green Tea

½ of a cucumber

1 tablespoon of Aloe Vera gel

5 drops of Peppermint Essential Oil

Directions:

Brew one cup of Green tea using the Green tea bag and then place the tea in the refrigerator. While the tea is cooling, you will want to peel the ½ of a cucumber and puree it. Strain the pureed cucumber removing all of the solids. Discard the remaining solids that have been strained.

Once your Green tea has cooled, pour ¼ of a cup of the Green tea into your spray bottle, followed by 2 tablespoons of the pureed cucumber juice, 1 tablespoon of the Aloe Vera gel and up to 5 drops of the Peppermint Essential Oil. As with the other recipes, it is important for you to test the amount of Peppermint Essential oil as you add it, only adding one drop at a time.

Place the lid on the spray bottle and shake well. Place this in the refrigerator when not using. The tea will stay good for about 1 week.

The Green tea is packed with antioxidants that will help to repair your skin and soothe dry skin, which means that as you are cooling off, you will be treating your skin for sun damage, wrinkles, and fine lines as well.

9. Hydrating Face Mist

You will need:

1 cup of hot water

2 Green Tea Bags

4 drops of avocado oil

1 teaspoon of witch hazel

Directions:

Begin by steeping the tea bags in the hot water. After the tea has steeped, remove the tea bags and place the tea in the refrigerator. After the tea has cooled, you will pour it into your spray bottle, filling it ¾ of the way full. Add in the avocado oil and the witch hazel. Place the lid on the spray bottle and shake well.

Use the cooling spray several times a day, whenever you need a boost or cooling off, on your neck and your face.

The Green tea is going to help repair your skin while the avocado oil is going to help reduce the signs of aging and reduce dryness. The witch hazel is going to ensure that you do not have too much oil on your face and it is going to help to reduce acne.

10. Skin-Clearing Mist

You will need:

2 teaspoons of Himalayan Sea Salt

1 cup of Peppermint Tea

½ of a teaspoon of Tea Tree oil

3 drops of Lavender Essential oil

3 drops of Lemongrass Essential oil

Directions:

Begin by brewing the cup of Peppermint tea. While your Peppermint tea is still hot, you will want to add in the Himalayan Sea Salt and stir well to ensure that it dissolves.

After the tea is cooled, fill your spray bottle ¾ of the way full and then add in your Tea Tree oil, Lavender Essential oil, and the Lemongrass Essential oil. It is best to use a glass atomizer bottle because essential oils will degrade plastic bottles.

Place the lid on the bottle and shake well before each use. This is a great cooling spray that can be used after you have worked out in order to prevent breakouts and help cool you down. The Tea Tree oil in the spray, as well as the sea salt, are going to help treat any blemishes that you currently have and the lavender is going to help calm your mind while the lemongrass will lift your mood.

11. Cooling Toner Spray

You will need:

6 ounces of distilled water

3 bags of Hibiscus tea

1 ounce of witch hazel

½ of a teaspoon of vitamin C powder

Directions:

Begin by boiling the water. As soon as the water reaches a boil, turn the heat off and then add in the three bags of Hibiscus tea. Cover and allow the tea to steep for 20 minutes.

After 20 minutes, remove the tea bags from the tea and add in the witch hazel as well as the vitamin C powder. Stir well.

Transfer the mixture to a spray bottle and store in a cool, dry place for up to 2 weeks. Storing in the refrigerator will prolong the shelf life.

Before using this on your face, you will want to apply it to your neck to ensure you have no sensitivities. Use this cooling toning spray each morning and each evening.

The Hibiscus Tea is going to help to cleanse and tone the skin while balancing the pH levels of the skin. Hibiscus Tea is going to tighten the skin without stripping the skin of its natural oils. The Vitamin C is going to help fight the signs of aging and the witch hazel is going to help dry up any excess oil, all while cooling your skin.

12. Cucumber Cool Down

You will need:

1/3 of a cup of distilled water

30 drops of Cucumber Seed oil

4 tablespoons of Aloe Vera Oil

Directions:

Place all of the ingredients into your spray bottle, place the lid on the spray bottle and shake well. This spray is going to separate so it is important for you to shake it each time you use it.

Chapter 3 – Calm Down, Cool Down, Sleep Tight Cooling Sprays and More

13. *Calm Down Cooling Spray*

You will need:

3 tablespoons Rosewater

3 tablespoons Witch Hazel

Distilled water

3 drops of Peppermint Essential Oil

Directions:

Begin by placing the 3 drops of Peppermint Essential oil in the bottle. Then fill the bottle 1/3 of the way full with distilled water. Next, you will add in the rose water and the witch hazel.

Place the lid on the spray bottle and shake well. This is a great spray for not only when you need to cool down, but for when you need to calm down as well.

14. *Sleep Tight Cooling Spray*

You will need:

30 drops of Lavender Essential oil

10 drops of Orange Essential Oil

Distilled water

2 drops of Peppermint Essential Oil

Directions:

Begin by placing all of the essential oils into your spray bottle and then fill the rest of the way with the distilled water. Place the lid on the spray bottle and shake well.

This is a great cooling spray to use on those nights when you are just too hot to go to sleep or for hot flashes that you get at night. It will not only cool you but it will relax you enough so that you will be able to fall asleep quickly.

15. Soothing Aloe and Lavender Mist

You will need:

Distilled water

30 drops of Lavender Essential oil

1 tablespoon of Rose Hip Essential oil

Aloe Vera Juice

Directions:

Begin by filling your spray bottle ¾ of the way full with the distilled water. Add in the Lavender Essential oil and the Rose Hip Essential oil. Fill the bottle the rest of the way with the Aloe Vera Juice.

Place the lid on the spray bottle and shake it well. Before you use this on your face, you will want to make sure that there is nothing in it that will cause you any irritation. Lavender can cause some people's skin to become irritated so it is important for you to do a patch test on your wrist before you put it on your face.

16. Rosewater Cooling Mist

You will need:

Rosewater

5 drops of Evening Primrose oil

1 drop of Peppermint Essential Oil

Directions:

Begin by placing the Peppermint Essential oil in your spray bottle followed by the Evening Primrose oil. Fill the bottle the rest of the way with the rosewater. Place the lid on the spray bottle and shake well.

This is a great cooling spray that will also benefit the skin. The rosewater is going to help to calm any inflammation while hydrating the skin. When you add in the Evening Primrose oil, you are going to find that the mist has a very sweet smell that can be used instead of perfume.

17. Energizing Cooling Mist

If you find that you have hit the midday slump, instead of reaching for another cup of coffee, reach for this cooling mist that is not only sweet smelling but that will energize you as well.

The Aloe Vera in the spray is going to help to cool your skin as well as soothe any irritated areas, while the sweet almond and the macadamia oil are going to help hydrate your skin and the coconut water is going to help energize you.

You will need:

Coconut water

Aloe Vera gel

1 tablespoon of Sweet Almond Essential Oil

1 tablespoon of Macadamia Essential oil

Directions:

Begin by placing the 1 tablespoon of the Sweet Almond Essential oil in your spray bottle as well as the 1 tablespoon of Macadamia Essential oil. Next, fill the bottle ½ of the way with the coconut oil and then finish filling the bottle with the Aloe Vera gel.

It is important for you to know that Coconut Water will go bad so it is important for you to place this spray in the refrigerator and to use it within 7 days. If you do not want to do this, you can replace the coconut oil with regular water but you will be giving up the benefits of the coconut oil.

18. Refreshing Cooling Mist

You will need:

Distilled water

Witch Hazel

10 drops of Neroli and Avocado Essential oil blend

Directions:

Begin by placing the 10 drops of the essential oil blend in the spray bottle. Next, fill the bottle ¾ of the way full with the distilled water and then fill it the rest of the way with the witch hazel.

Place the lid on the spray bottle and shake well. This is a great blend for those that have oily skin or those that suffer from acne. The witch hazel is going to help improve the pores while the spray cools your skin.

Chapter 4- More Amazing Cooling Sprays

19. Creating Your Own Cooling Spray

You will need:

Your favorite essential oils (8-20 drops each)

½ of a teaspoon of vodka

½ of a teaspoon of Aloe Vera Gel

½ of a teaspoon of glycerin

½ of a teaspoon of witch hazel extract

4 drops of Peppermint Essential Oil

Distilled water

Directions:

The first thing that you are going to want to do is to choose which essential oils you will use. In order to do this, you will take the caps off of all of your essential oils and then begin smelling them in pairs. Once you find a few that you like, smell them with your Peppermint essential oil.

After you have determined what essential oils you will use, add between 8 and 20 drops of each to your spray bottle, do not add the Peppermint Essential oil yes.

Next, you will add in the vodka, Aloe Vera gel, glycerin, and witch hazel extract to the bottle. Place the lid on the bottle and shake well. Take the lid off of the bottle and fill it the rest of the way with the distilled water. Finally, begin adding in the

Peppermint Essential oil, testing your cooling spray until you are happy with the effects.

The Aloe Vera is going to help soothe the skin, the witch hazel will help to treat any inflammation or acne, the vodka is going to work as an astringent and the peppermint is going to help cool the skin.

This spray is going to work as a light perfume, facial toner, cooling spray, and skin soother.

20. Rose Cooling Spray and Toner

You will need:

3 tablespoons of Rose Hydrosol

1 tablespoon of glycerin

1 tablespoon of witch hazel

Directions:

Place all of the ingredients into a spray bottle and shake well. It is important for you to make sure that you shake the bottle each time you apply the spray. It can be used on both your body and your face. The spray is a great toner, skin refresher and cooler that can be used during the summer months.

21. Super Effective Cooling Spray

You will need:

3 tablespoons of Aloe Vera gel

3 tablespoons of Witch Hazel

5 drops of Peppermint Essential Oil

Directions:

Place all of the ingredients into your spray bottle and shake well. Use this on your face, neck, feet, and wrists. If you are extremely hot, spray this on your face and then let the breeze blow on you to cool you even more. You can store this spray for up to three months in a cool, dark and dry place.

22. Chamomile Mist

You will need:

1 cup of strongly brewed Chamomile tea that has cooled

¼ of a cup of Aloe Vera Juice

10 drops of Lavender Essential oil

Directions:

After the tea has cooked, you will pour it into your spray bottle, then add in the Aloe Vera juice and the essential oil. Place the lid on the bottle and shake well. This is a great cooling spray for sunburns.

23. Refreshing and Cooling Spray

You will need:

3 tablespoons of Aloe Vera Gel

3 tablespoons of Witch Hazel

3 tablespoons of Cranberry Juice

2 tablespoons of distilled water

1 tablespoon of vegetable glycerin

3 drops Tangerine Essential oil

1 drop Ginger essential oil

Directions:

Begin by placing all of the ingredients in a bowl and mixing them well. After the ingredients are completely mixed, pour them into your spray bottle and place the lid on the bottle. Shake this mixture before using and store in a dark, cool area.

24. Lavender and Chamomile Cooling Spray

You will need:

3 ounces of strongly brewed Chamomile Tea

1 ½ ounces of Aloe Vera Gel

13 drops of Lavender Essential oil

Directions:

Begin by placing the Lavender Essential oil in the spray bottle followed by the Aloe Vera gel and then add in the Chamomile tea. Place the lid on the bottle and shake well.

25. Summer Cooling Spray

You will need:

1 drop Peppermint essential oil

3 drops Palmarosa essential oil

3 drops Lime essential oil

3 drops Grapefruit Essential oil

3 drops Geranium Essential oil

4 ounces of Aloe Vera Gel

Directions:

Place all of the ingredients in your spray bottle. Place the lid on the spray bottle and shake well before each use.

26. Peppermint Herb Cooling Spray

You will need:

1 tablespoon of loose peppermint herb or one bag of peppermint tea

1 cup of water

5 drops of Peppermint essential oil

13 drops of Lavender essential oil

1 tablespoon of Aloe Vera gel

10 drops of Tea Tree oil

Directions:

Begin by making a hot herbal infusion using either the tea bag or loose herbs. If you use loose herbs, strain the tea after it has steeped in order to remove the herbs.

Put the essential oils into the spray bottle as well as the Aloe Vera gel and then fill the rest of the way with the tea. Shake well. Refrigerate between uses to prolong the shelf life.

27. Ylang Lime Cooling Body Spray

You will need:

2 drops of Ylang Ylang essential oil

10 drops of Lime Essential Oil

2 tablespoons of vodka

Directions:

Mix all of the ingredients in your spray bottle and shake well before using.

28. Lavender and Lime Cooling Body Spray

You will need:

2 tablespoons of vodka

3 drops of Lavender essential oil

8 drops of Lime Essential Oil

Directions:

Mix all of the ingredients in your spray bottle and shake well before using.

29. Super Energizing Cooling Spray

You will need:

Distilled water

1 tablespoon of witch hazel

15 drops of Grapefruit essential oil

5 drops of Lavender essential oil

Directions:

Begin by placing the essential oils in the spray bottle followed by the witch hazel. Next, fill the spray bottle the rest of the way full with the distilled water. Place the lid on the spray bottle and shake well before using.

30. Cooling and Comforting Spray

You will need:

Distilled water

1 tablespoon of witch hazel

10 drops of Cinnamon Leaf essential oil

15 drops of Sweet Orange essential oil

Directions:

Begin by placing the essential oils in the spray bottle followed by the witch hazel. Next, fill the spray bottle the rest of the way full with the distilled water. Place the lid on the spray bottle and shake well before using.

Chapter 5- Even More Cooling Sprays

31. Brain Power Increasing Cooling Spray

You will need:

Distilled water

1 tablespoon of witch hazel

10 drops of Peppermint Essential Oil

15 drops of Patchouli essential oil

Directions:

Begin by placing the essential oils in the spray bottle followed by the witch hazel. Next, fill the spray bottle the rest of the way full with the distilled water. Place the lid on the spray bottle and shake well before using.

32. After Sun Cooling Spray

You will need:

4 ounces of Aloe Vera Gel

15 drops of Lavender essential oil

1 ounce of Vitamin E oil

5 drops of Eucalyptus essential oil

5 tablespoons of witch hazel

5 tablespoons of distilled water

Directions:

Place all of the ingredients into your spray bottle and shake well before each use. Use this spray after you have spent the day in the sun to reduce your chances of burning, cool, soothe, and moisturize the skin. Using this will help you get the sun-kissed look on your skin instead of the boiled lobster look.

33. Orange Blossom Cooling Spray

You will need:

1 ounce of distilled water

60 drops of Orange essential oil

½ of a teaspoon of vegetable glycerin

Directions:

Mix all of the ingredients in your spray bottle, place the lid on the spray bottle, and shake well before each use.

34. Bohemian Patchouli Body Spray

You will need:

1 ounce of distilled water

1/8 of a teaspoon of Tunisian Patchouli essential oil

½ of a teaspoon of vegetable glycerin

Directions:

Mix all of the ingredients in your spray bottle, place the lid on the spray bottle, and shake well before each use.

35. Menopause Cooling Spray

You will need:

1 tablespoon of dried peppermint

2 tablespoons of dried sage

½ of a cup of boiling water

2 tablespoons of witch hazel extract

1 ½ teaspoons of vegetable glycerin

½ teaspoon of Aloe Vera gel

3 drops of Lavender essential oil

3 drops of Rose Geranium essential oil

3 drops of Peppermint Essential Oil

1 4-ounce spray bottle

Directions:

Add the sage and peppermint to your boiling water and allow to steep until the water has completely cooled. Strain the loose herbs out of the tea.

Place all of the ingredients into your spray bottle and place the lid on the bottle. Shake vigorously. Shake this mixture before each use.

Chapter 6- A Few Tips for Making Body Sprays

There are a few things that you need to know when you are making your own body sprays, whether they be cooling body sprays or if you are making them simply for the fragrance.

1. You will want to make several body sprays because just as you have different perfumes for your different moods and activities, you will want different body sprays.

2. Always shake the bottle before using your newly made body sprays because oil and water will separate when they are left to sit.

3. Check the ingredient label on the products that your body sprays out of. You want to get organic, natural products that are not packed full of chemicals that can irritate the skin.

4. When you are using essential oils to create your body sprays, it is important that you purchase glass spray bottles because essential oils will degrade the plastic bottles over time. These can be purchased online for a fairly good price.

5. If you are using vodka or witch hazel in your body sprays, they are going to have a longer shelf life, lasting up to a few months, however, never add vodka to mists that you are putting on a sunburn. If you do use vodka in sprays that you will use on your face, make sure that you do not get it in your eyes.

If you are afraid of getting the cooling sprays or body sprays that you create in your eyes, simply use a washcloth and dab the cooling spray onto your skin.

6. If you are not using alcohol in your cooling mists or body sprays, you will want to store it in the fridge because it can go badly very quickly.

7. You can use an emulsifier in your sprays such as polysorbate 20 which will help the water and oil mix together, giving the product consistency and it will help to preserve the product which is important if you are giving it as a gift.

8. Be very careful when you are spraying body sprays that contain essential oils or any other oil that you do not get them on your clothes as they will stain.

Conclusion

There are so many different benefits that you can get from all of the cooling sprays that are found in this book. Not only are you able to cool your body on those hot summer days, while you are at work, or while you are experiencing hot flashes, but you can also benefit from the cooling spray in many other ways.

Each of these cooling sprays provides you with many different benefits, some of them will provide you with anti aging benefits, reduce acne, soothe inflammation, help you relax, increase your focus and much more.

Choose the cooling spray that you think you will benefit from the most or make several cooling sprays that you think you will enjoy. As you work through these body sprays, feel free to adjust the recipes and make them your own.

I hope that you have enjoyed this book and that you have found a few cooling sprays that will work for you and that you will enjoy making. Don't forget, these cooling sprays also work as perfumes and they are great gifts to give no matter what the season.

FREE Bonus Reminder

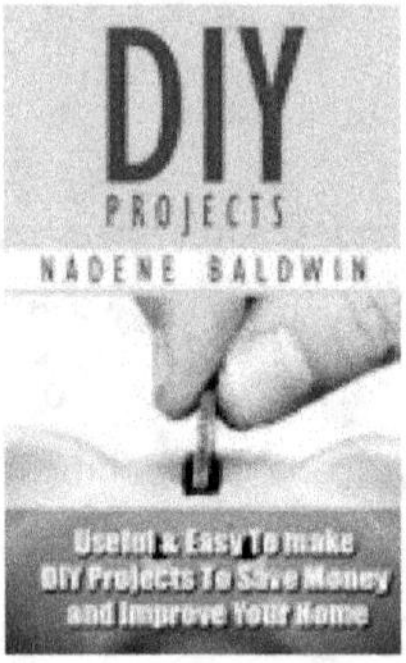

If you have not grabbed it yet, please go ahead and download your special bonus report *"DIY Projects. 13 Useful & Easy To Make DIY Projects To Save Money & Improve Your Home!"*

Simply Click the Button Below

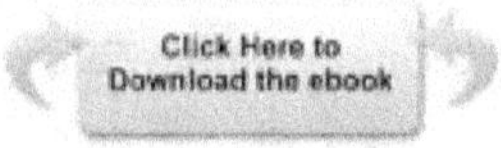

OR **Go to This Page**

http://diyhomecraft.com/free

BONUS #2: More Free & Discounted Books or Products

Do you want to receive more Free/Discounted Books or Products?

We have a mailing list where we send out our new Books or Products when they go free or with a discount on Amazon. Click on the link below to sign up for Free & Discount Book & Product Promotions.

=> Sign Up for Free & Discount Book & Product Promotions <=

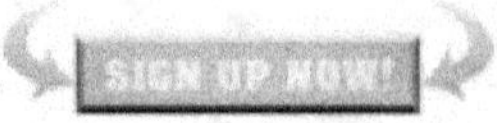

OR Go to this URL

http://zbit.ly/1WBb1Ek

www.ingramcontent.com/pod-product-compliance
Lightning Source LLC
Chambersburg PA
CBHW061324250726

48657CB00003B/1036